Contents

What Is A "Blue Zone" Diet?

"Blue Zone" is a non-scientific term given to geographic regions that are home to some of the world's oldest people.

In the early 2000s, Dan Buettner embarked on a mission to determine what specific aspects of lifestyle and environment help humans live longer. He teamed up with National Geographic and the National Institute of Aging on his quest, and through research, they were able to identify five areas with the highest percentage of centenarians (i.e. a person who is 100 years old or older). Known as the Blue Zones, these areas also have low rates of chronic diseases including heart disease, diabetes, and cancer. Buettner and his team of anthropologists, epidemiologists, and researchers traveled to these particular areas to study the lifestyle characteristics of the people who lived in these Blue Zones. From there, the "Blue Zone" diet became of interest to help people outside of these locations practice that way of life. Here's everything you need to know about the Blue Zones, including diet recommendations and more.

What are the five specific locations of the Blue Zones?

1. Sardinia, Italy: Sardinia is the second-largest island in the Mediterranean Sea and home to some of the world's longest-living males. The local shepherds walk at least five mountainous miles daily and follow a predominately plant-based diet. Meat is enjoyed on Sundays and special occasions only.

2. Okinawa, Japan: The world's longest-living women are from Okinawa, a chain of islands in Japan. Their longevity is suggested to be in part due to their close-knit social circles, as well as an old Confucian mantra said before meals that reminds them to avoid overeating and stop when they are 80% full.

3. Loma Linda, California: The residents of this city in San Bernardino have one of the highest rates of longevity in America. The community of Seven-Day Adventists in Loma Linda follow a primarily vegan diet and also recognize their Sabbath day weekly.

4. Nicoya, Costa Rica: The Nicoya Peninsula is known for elders with a positive outlook on life. Their diet is abundant in tropical fruits packed

with antioxidants, and their water is rich in calcium and magnesium that helps to prevent heart disease and builds strong bones.

5. Ikaria, Greece: This island in Greece is known for the long-living locals who embrace a Mediterranean diet abundant in olive oil, fruits, vegetables, whole grains, and beans. Ikarians also take time for a mid-afternoon break. They experience half the rate of heart disease and 20% less cancer than Americans do. Additionally, most Ikarians are Greek Orthodox Christians that follow several periods of fasting throughout the year where they essentially follow a vegan diet.

What habits contribute to the Blue Zone lifestyle?

Although the Blue Zones are all over the world, they share quite a few commonalities. After studying the Blue Zone populations, Buettner and his team narrowed down nine evidence-based common denominators among all of the world's centenarians. Known as the "Power 9," these factors are said to be the most influential in promoting longevity in these Blue Zone groups.

1. Move naturally: Centenarians don't run marathons or frequent the heavy lifting section of the gym. Instead, they are just constantly active throughout the day by tending to their gardens, cooking, doing house work, and

walking. Research on Sardinian men specifically found that residing in mountainous areas, walking longer distances to work, and shepherding are linked to their longevity.

2. Purpose: Blue Zone natives have a keen sense of purpose which motivates them in every day life. Ikigai and plan de vida are phrases from the Okinawans and Nicoyans, respectively, and both translate to, "why I wake up in the morning."

3. Downshift: Stress is inevitable wherever you live, but centenarians take time each day to de-stress whether it's praying, taking a nap, or enjoying a glass of wine.

4. Eighty percent rule: The Okinawan phrase hara hachi bu is said before meals to remind Okinawans to stop eating when they are 80%

full. This plays a role in weight management as well and fighting off obesity.

5. Plant slant: Fresh produce, especially homegrown, and beans are the cornerstones of most diets of Blue Zone people. On average, meat is only eaten five times per month in the Blue Zone regions.

6. Wine: Most Blue Zone people, except Adventists, drink 1 to 2 glasses of wine per day with friends or at a meal. Sardinian Cannonau wine, made from Grenache grapes, specifically has significantly more healthy flavonoids than other wines. Tea is also sipped daily throughout the Blue Zone regions, but beverages like soft drinks are practically unknown.

7. Faith: The vast majority of Blue Zone people belong to a faith-based community and attend faith-based services regularly.

8. Family: Centenarians put family first and are all about keeping the family close. They commit to a life partner and take time to build memories with their children.

9. Social networks: Friendship and close social circles support healthy behaviors in the Blue Zone regions. Okinawans in particular have created something called moais, which are groups of five friends that are committed to each other for life.

How does it work?

Research suggests that a strong mechanism behind the longevity and reduction of chronic disease in Blue Zone people is the anti-inflammatory benefits of their dietary choices. While these centenarians aren't necessarily completely vegan, their diets do have a predominant focus on plants.

Vegetables, especially homegrown, are a huge emphasis for Blue Zone people and provide a ton of vitamins, minerals, fiber, and antioxidant benefits. Beans and lentils are strong plant-based sources of protein in these populations. Similarly to vegetables, legumes also provide a ton of fiber which has benefits ranging from reducing risk of cardiovascular disease to helping control blood sugar levels. Healthy fats, such as olive oil, are used in several of the Blue Zone regions and provide a slew of heart-healthy fatty acids and antioxidants.

Blue zone people limit their consumption of red meat, and even only enjoy small portions of fish about three times per week. These populations do still indulge in moderation regarding sweets and other foods, but they eat sensibly and don't overindulge. By maintaining moderation and balance with food choices, especially following rules such as the Okinawans do with the hara hachi bu principle, weight stays controlled and obesity is not as prevalent to fuel chronic disease.

Foods in the Blue Zone Diet

The Blue Zone diet includes:

• Fruits and vegetables. "They're a great source of fiber and many different vitamins and minerals," DeRobertis says. Eating more than five servings of fruits and vegetables a day can significantly reduce your risk of heart disease, cancer and death.

• Legumes. Legumes include beans, peas, lentils and chickpeas, and they are all rich in fiber and protein. "A number of studies have shown that eating legumes is associated with lower mortality," DeRobertis says.

• Whole grains. A high intake of whole grains, which are also rich in fiber, can reduce blood pressure and is associated with reduced colorectal cancer and death from heart disease.

• Nuts. "Nuts are great sources of fiber, protein and polyunsaturated and monounsaturated fats," DeRobertis says. "Combined with a healthy diet, they're associated with reduced mortality and may even help reverse metabolic syndrome."

• Fish. Often eaten in Icaria and Sardinia, fish is a good source of omega-3 fats, which are important for heart and brain health.

Blue Zones people also follow reduced calorie intake and fasting. Long-term calorie restriction may help longevity, DeRobertis says. "A large, 25-year study in monkeys found that eating 30% fewer calories than normal led to a significantly longer life. Studies in the Okinawans suggest that before the 1960s, they were in a calorie deficit, meaning that they were eating fewer calories than they required, which may be contributing to their longevity," she says. "Okinawans tend to follow the 80% rule, which they call hara hachi bu. This means that they stop eating when they feel 80% full, rather than 100% full. This prevents them from eating too many calories, which can lead to weight gain and chronic disease."

In addition, people in some Blue Zones drink one to two glasses of red wine per day, which may help prevent heart disease and reduce the risk of death. And while people in these zones don't exercise in a gym, "activity is built into their daily lives through gardening, walking, cooking and other daily chores," DeRobertis says.

Blue Zone diet food list:

Based on the "Power 9" principle of plant slant that the Blue Zone regions embrace, we've put together a food list that can help you get started on eating the Blue Zone way.

Produce

- Fruit: apples, bananas, berries, grapes, oranges, papaya, pineapple, plums, watermelon, etc

- Vegetables: bell peppers, beets, broccoli, carrots, cauliflower, chard, collard greens, cucumber, garlic, green beans, kale, onions, potatoes, spinach, tomatoes, etc.

Protein

- Beans & legumes: black beans, chickpeas, kidney beans, lentils, etc.
- Eggs (up to two to four times per week)

- Fish (up to three small servings a week): anchovies, salmon, cod, swordfish, tuna, sardines, etc.

- Goat milk and goat-based dairy products

- Nuts: almonds, Brazil nuts, cashews, peanuts, walnuts, etc.

- Seeds: pumpkin seeds, chia seeds, flax seeds, hemp seeds, etc.

- Tofu, extra-firm

Grains & Pantry Staples

- Barley

- Brown Rice

- Coffee

- Dried spices and fresh herbs

- Oatmeal, preferably steel-cut

- Olive oil

- Quinoa

- Red wine

- Tea

- 100% Whole wheat, sprouted grain bread, and sourdough bread

7 Blue Zone Foods to Include in Your Diet

For a long life and better health, try boosting your intake of foods that people living in Blue Zones have in their diet. A concept developed by National Geographic Fellow and author Dan

Buettner, Blue Zones are areas across the globe where people tend to live the longest and have remarkably low rates of heart disease, cancer, diabetes, and obesity.

With their strikingly high concentrations of individuals who live to be over 100-years-old, Blue Zones include the following regions: Ikaria, Greece; Okinawa, Japan; the province of Ogliastra in Sardinia, Italy; the community of Seventh-Day Adventists in Loma Linda, California; and Costa Rica's Nicoya Peninsula.

A wholesome diet isn't the only factor thought to lead to longevity for those living in Blue Zones, however. Such individuals also have high levels of physical activity, low stress levels, robust social connections, and a strong sense of purpose.1

Still, sticking to a vibrant, nutrient-rich eating plan appears to play a key role in the exceptional health of Blue Zone dwellers. Here's a look at seven foods to include in your own Blue Zone-inspired diet.

1. Legumes

From chickpeas to lentils, legumes are a vital component of all Blue Zone diets.1 Loaded with fiber and known for their heart-healthy effects, legumes also serve as a top source of protein, complex carbohydrates, and a variety of vitamins and minerals.

Whether you prefer pinto beans or black-eyed peas, aim for at least a half-cup of legumes each day. Ideal for any meal, legumes make a great addition to salads, soups and stews, and many veggie-based recipes.

"If you want to make a three-bean chili for dinner, use dry beans and soak them, cooking them with your own spices and fresh veggies," recommends registered dietician Maya Feller, owner of Maya Feller Nutrition.

2. Dark Leafy Greens

While vegetables of all kinds abound in each Blue Zone diet, dark leafy greens like kale, spinach, and Swiss chard are especially prized. One of the most nutrient-dense types of veggies, dark leafy greens contain several vitamins with powerful antioxidant properties, including vitamin A and vitamin C.

3. Nuts

Like legumes, nuts are packed with protein, vitamins, and minerals. They also supply heart-healthy unsaturated fats, with some research suggesting that including nuts in your diet may help reduce your cholesterol levels (and, in turn, stave off cardiovascular disease).

"Nuts are a high-fiber food," says Feller. "Almonds, for instance, provide about 3.5 grams of fiber in a one-ounce serving." For healthier snacking, borrow a habit from Blue Zone residents and try a handful of almonds, walnuts, pistachios, cashews, or Brazil nuts.

4. Olive Oil

A staple of Blue Zone diets, olive oil offers a wealth of health-enhancing fatty acids, antioxidants, and compounds such as oleuropein (a chemical found to curb inflammation).

Select the extra-virgin variety of olive oil as often as possible, and use your oil for cooking and in salads and vegetable dishes. Olive oil is sensitive to light and heat, so be sure to store it in a cool, dark area like a kitchen cabinet.

5. Steel-Cut Oatmeal

When it comes to whole grains, those in Blue Zones often choose oats. One of the least processed forms of oats, steel-cut oats make for a high-fiber and incredibly filling breakfast option.

Although they're perhaps best known for their cholesterol-lowering power, oats may also provide plenty of other health benefits. For instance, recent research has determined that oats may thwart weight gain, fight diabetes, and prevent hardening of the arteries.

"Oats are known for their fiber content, but they also provide plant-based protein," says Feller. "Oatmeal made with 1/4 cup of steel-cut oats provides 7 grams of protein."

6. Blueberries

Fresh fruit is the go-to sweet treat for many people living in Blue Zones. While most any type of fruit can make for a healthy dessert or snack, foods such as blueberries may offer bonus benefits.

For example, recent studies have demonstrated that blueberries may help shield your brain health as you age.6 But the benefits might go even further. Other research says blueberries might fend off heart disease by improving blood pressure control.

7. Barley

Another whole grain favored in Blue Zones, barley may possess cholesterol-lowering properties similar to those of oats, according to a study published in the European Journal of

Clinical Nutrition. Barley also delivers essential amino acids, as well as compounds that may help stimulate digestion.

To get your fill of barley, try adding this whole grain to soups or consuming it as a hot cereal.

Achieving A Blue Zone Benefit

If you're interested in adding years to your life, you don't have to move to a Blue Zone or adopt a vegetarian diet. The idea is to incorporate as many of the Power 9 tenets as possible into your busy life.

"People in Blue Zones eat more plant-based foods, fewer processed foods, they spend less time on devices, they move as part of their daily repertoire, and they value family, faith, and community," says Conley. "They also find time to unwind."

BLUE ZONE DIET RECIPES

Trying blue zone-friendly recipes is a great way to explore new flavors and find new favorite dishes while looking after your health. In this part are nourishing blue zone diet recipes for you to enjoy.

Blueberry Muffin Energy Bites

Preparation time

10 minutes

INGREDIENTS

- 1 cup old fashioned rolled oats or quick oats

- ½ cup dried blueberries

- 1 tablespoon chia seeds

- ¾ almond butter

- 2 tablespoons pure maple syrup

- ¼ teaspoon cinnamon

- Pinch of salt

Instructions

1. In a large bowl, stir together all ingredients until well combined.

2. Roll into 12-14 balls.

3. Store in an airtight container in the fridge.

No-Egg Eggnog

Preparation time

3 hours

INGREDIENTS

- ½ cup raw cashews, soaked in water overnight

or for at least 4 hours, drained, and rinsed

- 1 cup water

- 1 cup full-fat coconut cream

- 1 cup unsweetened, plain soy milk

- 2½ tablespoons granulated sugar

- 1½ teaspoons vanilla extract

- 1 teaspoon ground cinnamon

- ¼ teaspoon ground nutmeg

- ⅛ teaspoon ground cloves

- ⅛ teaspoon ground cardamom

Instructions

1. In a high-powered blender, combine the soaked cashews, water, coconut cream, soy milk, sugar, vanilla extract, cinnamon, cloves, and cardamom and purée until smooth.

2. Place the nog in the refrigerator and chill for 2 to 3 hours.

3. Stir the nog and serve cold.

Creamy Pumpkin Marinara Pasta

Preparation time

20 minutes

INGREDIENTS

- 1 box rotini

- 2 tablespoons olive oil

- 2 garlic cloves, minced

- ½ yellow onion, diced

- ½ teaspoon oregano

- ¼ teaspoon cinnamon

- ½ teaspoon salt

- 1 can crushed tomatoes

- ½ can pumpkin puree

- ½ cup vegetable broth

- Fresh basil

- ¼ cup parmesan, shredded (optional)

Instructions

1. Cook rotini pasta according to instructions.

2. Drain and set aside.

3. Add oil to a large pot over medium heat and sauté onion until tender.

4. Add garlic and sauté for another minute.

5. Add pumpkin, tomato, broth, and seasonings.

6. Bring to a boil and stir continuously for about 10 minutes.

7. In a large mixing bowl, toss pasta with sauce and divide into two servings.

8. Serve pasta with fresh grated cheese and garnish with basil.

Classic Stuffed Shells

Preparation time

1 hour

INGREDIENTS

- 1 (12-ounce) package jumbo pasta shells

- 1 (16-ounce) block firm (or extra-firm) tofu, pressed

- 1 medium yellow onion, roughly chopped

- 5 medium cloves garlic

- ¼ cup packed fresh basil leaves

- 2 teaspoons dried oregano

- 2 teaspoons salt

- ¾ teaspoon ground black pepper

- ¼ teaspoon red chili pepper flakes (optional)

- 2 tablespoons nutritional yeast

- Juice of 1 medium lemon

- 1 cup packed spinach leaves

- 1 (25-ounce) jar flavorful marinara sauce, divided

- ½ cup vegan cheese shreds (optional)

- Fresh basil leaves, for garnish (optional)

Instructions

1. In a large pot of boiling water, cook the jumbo pasta shells according to the prebake cooking directions on the package.

2. Then drain, rinse with cold water to prevent sticking, and set aside.

3. Meanwhile, in the bowl of a food processor, combine the tofu, onion, garlic, basil, oregano, salt, black pepper, red chili pepper flakes (if

using), nutritional yeast, and lemon juice. Pulse 15 times or until partially mixed.

4. Add the spinach and pulse just a few more times until combined. The resulting texture should be ricotta-like. Do not over pulse or your ricotta will turn green!

5. Preheat the oven to 375 degrees F.

6. Pour half of the marinara sauce into a 9 × 13-inch baking dish, spreading to evenly coat the bottom of the dish.

7. One by one, fill each cooked shell with a generous spoonful of the tofu ricotta filling and place in the prepared baking dish.

8. Continue until the tofu mixture is gone and the baking dish is filled.

9. Sprinkle the vegan cheese (if using) on top.

10. Drizzle the remaining marinara sauce over the stuffed shells.

11. Cover the pan with aluminum foil and bake for 20 minutes.

12. Remove the foil and bake for another 20 minutes or until the cheese (if using) is melted and the edges of the shells are lightly browned.

13. Garnish with the basil leaves (if using).

14. Serve immediately and enjoy hot.

Classic Stuffing

Preparation time

1 hour 25 minutes

INGREDIENTS

- 1 (16-ounce) loaf French bread

- 2 cups vegetable broth (or equivalent amount of vegetable bouillon and water)

- 1 tablespoon ground flaxseed meal

- ½ cup vegan butter, plus additional for greasing the dish

- 3 medium ribs celery, diced

- 1 medium yellow onion, diced

- 1 medium Granny Smith apple, cored and finely diced

- ⅓ cup finely chopped fresh parsley

- 2 teaspoons poultry seasoning

Instructions

1. Cut the bread loaf into small (bite-sized) cubes, spread the bread cubes across a large baking sheet, and leave them out overnight or for at least 12 hours. The next day, preheat the oven to 250 degrees F and bake for 30 minutes to fully dry out the bread. Grease a 9 × 13-inch baking dish with vegan butter. Transfer the dried bread cubes to the prepared baking dish and set aside.

2. In a medium bowl, whisk together the broth and flaxseed meal. Set aside for at least 10 minutes.

3. Preheat the oven to 375 degrees F.

4. In a medium pan over medium-high heat, melt the vegan butter. Add the celery, onion, and apple and sauté, mixing occasionally, for 5 minutes or until tender.

5. Pour the sautéed veggie mixture and the vegetable broth mixture evenly over the bread in the baking dish, and sprinkle evenly with the parsley and poultry seasoning. Using your hands, mix to evenly coat.

6. Cover with aluminum foil and bake for 40 minutes. Remove the foil and bake for another 40 minutes. Allow to cool for 15 minutes before serving.

Quick Pickled Vegetables

Preparation time

3-5 days

INGREDIENTS

- 1 bunch of turnips

- 1 bunch of radishes

- 1 Vidalia spring onion

- 1 cup of white vinegar

- 1 tablespoon of kosher salt

- 1 teaspoon pickling spice

- Red pepper flakes to taste

Instructions

For the brine:

1. Heat the vinegar, one cup of water, and kosher salt in a small saucepan, stirring until salt is fully dissolved.

2. Remove from heat.

3. Wash, stem and quarter the radishes and turnips.

4. Wash and thinly slice the Vidalia spring onions.

5. Separate into rings.

Assembly:

1. Divide the pickling spice and red pepper flakes in two wide-mouth, pint jars or glassworking jars with lids.

2. Arrange the turnips, radishes, and onion in each container.

3. Equally distribute the brine.

4. Cover and put in the fridge.

5. Quick pickles are ready between 3-5 days.

Ikarian Stuffed Eggplant (Imam Bayildi)

Preparation time

1 hour

INGREDIENTS

- 5 medium eggplants, ends cut off, scored deeply four times lengthwise

- 1 cup parsley, chopped

- 2 large tomatoes, diced

- 2 onions, diced

- 4 cloves garlic, sliced in thirds

- 1 cup extra-virgin olive oil

- 1 potato, peeled and thinly sliced

- 1 bell pepper (green, red, or yellow), diced

- Salt and pepper to taste

Instructions

1. In a large pan, sauté eggplants in olive oil for about 10 minutes, rotating often.

2. In a medium bowl, mix together parsley, tomatoes, onions, garlic, bell pepper, and 1 cup olive oil as your stuffing mixture.

3. In a separate pan, sauté stuffing for 6-8 minutes, or until onions are tender.

4. Add the stuffing mix on top and into the eggplants.

5. Place potatoes around the eggplants in the pan.

6. Cook over low heat for about 30 minutes, checking the pan for liquid and basting with cooking liquid, if needed.

BBQ Jackfruit Sandwiches

Preparation time

15 minutes

INGREDIENTS

- 1 batch BBQ Pulled Jackfruit

- 1 cup finely shredded purple cabbage (or coleslaw, store-bought or from the recipe on page 162)

- 1 large red onion, finely sliced

- Dill pickles, sliced, to taste

- 4 burger buns, toasted

PULLED JACKFRUIT INGREDIENTS

- 2 (20-oz) cans young green jackfruit, drained

- 1 tbsp canola or vegetable oil

- ½ small red onion, diced

- 2 medium cloves garlic, minced

- 1 teaspoon smoked paprika

- 1 cup vegan barbecue sauce

DIRECTIONS

- Assemble each sandwich with a large scoop of hot BBQ pulled jackfruit topped with cabbage or coleslaw, red onion, and pickles on a toasted bun.

- Devour immediately.

Notes:

• Some brands of buns get soggy really easily. If that's a deal-breaker for you, try using a sturdier roll or ciabatta instead.

PULLED JACKFRUIT DIRECTIONS

• Using your fingers, pull apart the jackfruit pieces into shreds and remove all the tough pieces. Place the shreds and the oil in a medium pan

• Place the pan over medium-high heat and add the onion and garlic.

• Sauté for 4 minutes or until the onion becomes translucent.

• Add the paprika and cook for 3 more minutes.

- Pour in the barbecue sauce and cook for 3 minutes.

- Serve hot.

Roasted Potatoes & Green Beans with Mustard Drizzle

Preparation time

45 minutes

INGREDIENTS

- ½ pound fingerling potatoes

- 3 garlic cloves

- 3 tablespoons chopped fresh parsley or other herbs

- 2-3 tablespoons extra-virgin olive oil

- ½ cup cooked chickpeas (or canned, drained, and rinsed) patted dry with a paper towel

- ½ pound green beans

MUSTARD DRIZZLE DRESSING INGREDIENTS

- 1 tablespoon Dijon mustard

- 1½ tablespoons extra-virgin olive oil

- 1 tablespoon white wine vinegar

- 2 teaspoons honey

• Salt and pepper (optional)

Instructions

1. Heat oven to 425 degrees.

2. In a large mixing bowl, toss potatoes with garlic, herbs, and half of olive oil.

3. Place in a single layer in a roasting pan and roast for 25 minutes, stirring once or twice.

4. When potatoes are tender and starting to brown, add the chickpeas and green beans and roast for another 10 minutes.

5. While that roasts, in a small bowl whisk together mustard, olive oil, vinegar, and honey to form an emulsified dressing.

6. Season the dressing with salt and pepper to taste.

7. Transfer the roasted vegetables and beans to a platter and drizzle with dressing. Serve warm.

Instant Pot One-Pot Pasta with Cherry Tomatoes and Basil

Preparation time

40 minutes

INGREDIENTS

• 1 tablespoon extra virgin olive oil (optional), plus more to serve

- 1 small yellow onion, diced

- 4 cloves garlic, sliced

- ¼ teaspoon red pepper flakes

- 1 lb (450g) uncooked short pasta (such as penne, fusilli, or bowtie)

- 1 teaspoon sea salt

- 4–5 cups water

- 1 pint (551ml) cherry tomatoes

- 1 bunch fresh basil, torn or sliced

- ¼ cup drained capers

- 1 cup shredded vegan Parmesan cheese

- Freshly ground

Instructions

1. On the Instant Pot, select Sauté (Medium), and heat the oil, if using, in the inner pot until hot. (Otherwise, you can dry sauté in the hot pot or add a bit of water in the bottom of the pot.)

2. Add the onion and sauté until softened and golden, 3 to 5 minutes. Add the garlic and pepper and sauté 1 minute longer. Press Cancel.

3. Add the pasta to the inner pot of the Instant Pot.

4. Add the salt and water until just covered, no more than ¼ inch (0.5cm) above the pasta.

5. Add the tomatoes on top without stirring.

6. Lock the lid of the Instant Pot and ensure the steam release valve is set to the sealing position.

Select Pressure Cook (Low), and set the cook time for half of the cook time on the pasta package, rounding down. For example, if the pasta package calls for 10 to 12 minutes on the stove, set the cook time for 5 minutes.

7. Once the cook time is complete, immediately quick release the pressure and carefully remove the lid.

8. Add the fresh basil and capers, and stir to combine.

9. Drizzle with a little olive oil, if desired.

10. Serve immediately with Parmesan and salt and pepper, to taste.

11. Tip: If you're craving more protein, you can stir in a cup of cooked chickpeas or cannellini beans or serve with grilled vegan Italian

sausage. If you love greens, wilt in a few handfuls of arugula or spinach at the end.

French Lentils with Roasted Radishes

Preparation time

50 minutes

INGREDIENTS

- 1 ½ cups Puy (French) lentils, or black lentils

- 1 bay leaf

- Sea salt and ground black pepper

- 3 cups radishes

- 3 tablespoons olive oil, divided

- 3 large cloves garlic, pressed

- 2 tablespoons minced fresh mint

- ¼ cup minced fresh chives

- 3 tablespoons hemp seeds, divided

- 2 tablespoons fresh lemon juice

- 2 cups (packed) mâché or baby spinach

- ½ cup almond ricotta

Instructions

1. Preheat the oven to 450°F.

2. In a medium saucepan over high heat, combine the lentils and the bay leaf with about 5 cups of water. Bring to a boil, and then reduce the heat to medium-low.

3. Simmer gently until the lentils are tender but not mushy, about 15–20 minutes.

4. Drain the lentils in a colander over the sink, and remove the bay leaf.

5. Transfer the lentils to a bowl and season them with ½ teaspoon salt and ½ teaspoon ground black pepper.

6. Cover the bowl to keep the lentils warm.

7. Meanwhile, clean and trim the radishes, removing the stems, while leaving their tails intact. Halve the radishes lengthwise, and quarter any large halves.

8. Warm 1 tablespoon of the olive oil in an ovenproof saute pan* over medium-high heat.

9. When the oil is hot, add the radishes to the pan in a single layer (flat side down as much as possible), season generously with salt and pepper, and cook for 2–3 minutes to lightly sear the bottoms.

10. Remove the pan from the heat, stir in the garlic, distributing it well, and transfer the pan to the oven.

11. Roast the radishes for 7–12 minutes (depending on their size), until they are vibrantly red and lightly golden on the edges. Remove the pan from the oven.

12. In a large mixing bowl, combine the cooked lentils, roasted radishes and their cooking juices, and the remaining 2 tablespoons of olive oil.

13. Add the mint, chives, 2 tablespoons of the hemp seeds, lemon juice, and the mache or baby spinach to the bowl.

14. Toss the mixture to combine and season to taste with additional salt and pepper as desired.

15. Add the almond ricotta to the mixture in small dollops and fold it into the mixture gently, retaining the dollops as much as possible.

16. Sprinkle the remaining tablespoon of hemp seeds on top, and serve warm or at room temperature.

Instant Pot Quinoa Breakfast Bowls

Preparation time

30 minutes

INGREDIENTS

- 1 cup quinoa, rinsed and drained

- 1½ cups unsweetened almond or other plant-based milk, plus more to serve

- ½ teaspoon pure vanilla extract

- Pinch of ground cinnamon

FOR SERVING INGREDIENTS

- ¼ cup pure maple syrup

- 1 cup berries (any combination of blueberries, raspberries, or strawberries)

- 1 banana, sliced

- ½ cup slivered almonds, toasted

Instructions

1. In the inner pot, stir together the quinoa, almond milk, vanilla, and cinnamon. Lock the lid and ensure the steam release valve is set to the sealing position.

2. Select Pressure Cook (High), and set the cook time for 5 minutes.

3. Once the cook time is complete, immediately quick release the pressure.

4. Carefully remove the lid.

5. If desired, stir in more milk to thin into a porridge.

6. Serve warm in bowls, sweetened to taste with maple syrup and topped generously with fruit and almonds.

Spicy Eggplant with Garlic

Preparation time

20 minutes

INGREDIENTS

- ¼ cup vegetable broth

- 1 tablespoon soy sauce

- 1 tablespoon Chinese black vinegar or good balsamic vinegar

- 1 tablespoon brown sugar

- 1 tablespoon chili oil

- ¼ teaspoon red pepper flakes

- 2 tablespoons peanut or vegetable oil

- 2 to 3 Asian eggplants, cut into thin, 1-inch-long strips

- 2 scallions, minced

- 1 tablespoon fresh minced ginger

- 2 garlic cloves, minced

Instructions

1. In a small bowl, mix together the vegetable broth, soy sauce, vinegar, brown sugar, chili oil, and red pepper flakes. Set aside.

2. Place a wok over high heat until a drop of water sizzles on contact.

3. Add the peanut oil and swirl to coat the wok.

4. Add the eggplants to the wok, and stir-fry for 2 to 3 minutes, until the outsides become golden brown.

5. Turn down the heat to medium-high, and add the scallions, ginger, and garlic.

6. Stir-fry for about 30 seconds, and then add the broth mixture; toss the vegetables for 2 to 3 minutes until they are coated with the sauce.

7. Simmer the vegetables for 2 to 3 minutes, allowing the eggplant to absorb the sauce.

Matcha Custard With Berries

Preparation time

30 minutes

INGREDIENTS

- 1 cup raw cashews, soaked in water overnight

- 4 cups hot water

- 1 teaspoon matcha powder

- 7 tablespoons maple syrup

- 2 teaspoons vanilla extract

- ½ teaspoon sea salt

- 6 tablespoons arrowroot powder

- 1 ½ cups fresh blueberries or blackberries

Instructions

1. Rinse and drain cashews, then place in a blender.

2. Add hot water to blender, along with matcha powder.

3. If the top of your blender has a removable center cap, remove it to help release steam, and then cover the top with a kitchen towel.

4. Blend ingredients into a smooth milk.

5. Pour 1 cup of matcha milk into a medium bowl and set it aside.

6. Pour remaining matcha milk into a medium pot.

7. Whisk in maple syrup, vanilla extract, and salt.

8. Add arrowroot powder to reserved matcha milk in the bowl and whisk mixture into a slurry.

9. Add the slurry to matcha milk in the pot and warm it over medium-low heat.

10. Whisking continuously, cook mixture for 4–5 minutes or until it begins to thicken into a loose, pudding-like consistency.

11. Once the consistency has thickened, take the pot off the heat immediately—the custard will continue to solidify slightly as it cools.

12. Pour the custard into a large container or 6–8 individual small cups (ramekins work well).

13. Serve custard warm or cold, topped with plenty of fresh berries.

14. Brain-Boosting Optional Topping: Top each serving with 1/2 teaspoon cacao nibs.

Pantry-Style Spicy Street Noodles (Mee Goreng)

Preparation time

15 minutes

INGREDIENTS

- 1 tablespoon vegetable oil

- 1 small sweet onion, thinly sliced into strips

- 8 oz firm tofu, cut into strips (optional)

- 2 teaspoons minced garlic

- 2-3 cups chopped greens (spinach, bok choy, kale, mustard greens, shredded cabbage, green beans, or any combination of these)

- 12 oz fettuccine or rice noodles

- 1 teaspoon ground cumin

- 2-3 teaspoon sambal oelek or other sweet chili sauce like sriracha

- 3 tablespoons ketchup

- 2 tablespoons soy sauce

- Lemon for serving

Instructions

1. Cook noodles according to package directions.

2. Drain well.

3. Heat up a large pan or wok over high heat.

4. Add the oil, reduce heat to medium-high and saute the onion for 2-3 minutes.

5. Add garlic, greens, and tofu, if using, to pan and cook for another 3 minutes.

6. Mix spice and sauces in a bowl.

7. Add noodles to the pan, tossing and mixing with tongs or cooking chopsticks. (It's better if parts of the noodles get a bit crispy).

8. Add spice – sauce mixture and toss everything together.

9. Cook for another 2-3 minutes, until everything is combined and seasoned.

10. Transfer to individual serving bowls and serve with lemon wedges and sambal oelek.

Blueberry Chia Muffins

Preparation time

40 minutes

INGREDIENTS

- 1 ¾ cup spelt flour (whole wheat, gluten-free or whatever you have on hand will work just fine)

- 1 tablespoon baking powder

- ½ teaspoon sea salt

- ¾ teaspoon cinnamon

- ½ teaspoon cardamom

- 3 tablespoons chia seeds (1 teaspoon set aside for topping)

- 6 tablespoons coconut oil

- ¾ cup almond milk (oat milk, coconut milk, etc.)

- 7 tablespoons maple syrup

- 1 teaspoon vanilla extract

- 1 cup frozen blueberries

Instructions

1. Whisk dry ingredients.

2. Melt coconut oil on stovetop, mix in other wet ingredients over gentle heat until smooth.

3. Mix wet ingredients into dry ingredients.

4. Carefully stir in blueberries.

5. Scoop into muffin tin.

6. Sprinkle remaining chia seeds on top of muffins.

7. Bake in oven at 350 degrees F for 25-30 minutes.

Feel Better Noodle Soup

Preparation time

30 minutes

INGREDIENTS

- 1 tablespoon olive oil

- 2 yellow onions, diced

- 1 medium leek, sliced

- 8 cloves garlic, minced

- 1-inch knob of ginger, peeled and minced

- 6 cups vegetable broth

- 4 large carrots, peeled and chopped (about 2 cups)

- 5 stalks celery, chopped (about 2 cups)

- 2 tablespoons chopped fresh dill

- Salt and black pepper, to taste

Instructions

1. Prepare the pasta according to the instructions on the package.

2. Heat the olive oil in a large pot over medium heat.

3. Add the onions, leek, garlic, and ginger, and sauté for 5 minutes, until the onions are translucent.

4. Add the vegetable broth, carrots, celery, and dill, and bring to a simmer.

5. Cover the pot and simmer for 15–20 minutes, until the carrots and celery are tender.

6. Add the cooked pasta to the pot and season with salt and pepper.

7. Serve warm.

Take-Out Style Vegetable Lo Mein

Preparation time

20 minutes

INGREDIENTS

- 2 tablespoons soy sauce

- 2 teaspoons sugar

- 1 teaspoon sesame oil

- 1 teaspoon chili sauce (optional)

- 1 tablespoon peanut oil

- 2 garlic cloves, minced

- 1 ½ cups cremini or button mushrooms, sliced

- 1 red bell pepper, julienned

- ¼ cup shredded carrots

- ¼ cup shredded cabbage (red, green, or Napa)

- ½ cup snow peas

- 2 scallions, cut into 1-inch pieces

- ½ pound lo mein, cooked according to package directions

Instructions

1. In a small bowl, make the sauce by mixing the soy sauce, sugar, sesame oil, and chili sauce (if using). Set aside.

2. Heat your wok on high heat until a drop of water sizzles on contact.

3. Add the peanut oil and swirl to coat the wok.

4. Add garlic, cremini mushrooms, red bell pepper, and carrots to the wok, and stir-fry for 3 to 4 minutes, tossing often.

5. Add the snow peas and scallions, and stir-fry for another 2 to 3 minutes.

6. Add the lo mein and the sauce mixture to the wok.

7. Toss everything together to combine, and turn off the heat.

8. Serve immediately.

9. Note: If you don't have lo mein, you can make this with fettuccine, spaghetti, or even soba noodles with great results.

Paella with Chickpeas, Green Beans, and Shishito Peppers

Preparation time

30 minutes

INGREDIENTS

- 6 cups no-salt-added vegetable broth

- ¼ teaspoon crumbled saffron threads*

- 2 tomatoes, halved

- ½ cup extra-virgin olive oil

- 24 small shishito peppers, stemmed but left whole

- 1 large yellow onion, chopped

- 6 garlic cloves, chopped

- 2 red bell peppers, chopped

- 2 teaspoons Spanish smoked paprika (pimenton)

- 1 teaspoon ground cumin

- 1 teaspoon kosher salt, plus more to taste

- 1 pound fresh green beans, cut into 1-inch pieces

- ¼ cup finely chopped flat-leaf parsley leaves

- 3 cups imported Spanish rice, preferably Calasparra (may substitute Arborio)

- 3 cups cooked or canned no-salt-added chickpeas (from one 29-ounce can or two 15-ounce cans), drained and rinsed

- 2 cups spinach, chopped

- 1 cup Chickpea Aioli or store-bought vegan or traditional mayonnaise, mixed with 1 finely chopped garlic clove

Instructions

1. Preheat the oven to 400 º F.

2. In a saucepan, combine the broth and saffron over medium-high heat, bring to a boil, then reduce the heat to low and cover while you assemble the paella.

3. Set a box grater over a bowl and run the cut side of the tomatoes across the coarse side of the grater, continuing until you are left with just the skin.

4. Heat a 17-to 18-inch paella pan over two or three burners or heat two 10-to 11-inch cast-iron skillets over medium-high heat.

5. Pour in the olive oil and when it shimmers, add the shishitos, searing each side for a minute or two, then use tongs to transfer them to a plate.

6. Stir in the onion, garlic, and bell peppers and cook, stirring frequently, until the vegetables are soft, 6 to 8 minutes.

7. Stir in the paprika, cumin, and salt and cook until fragrant, about 30 seconds.

8. Stir in the green beans and cook, stirring frequently, until they lose a little of their crunch.

9. Stir in the tomato pulp and parsley and cook for about 30 seconds, then stir in the rice, coating it well with the pan mixture.

10. Stir in the broth, chickpeas, and spinach, taste, and add more salt if needed.

11. Cook, stirring and rotating the pan occasionally, until the mixture is no longer soupy, but the rice is still covered by liquid, about 5 minutes.

12. Nestle the shishitos on the rice and transfer the pan to the oven.

13. Bake, uncovered, until the rice is al dente, 12 to 15 minutes.

14. Remove, cover with aluminum foil, and let it sit for 10 minutes, until the rice is fully cooked.

15. Serve hot, with the aioli on the side.

Warm & Spicy Red Wine Wassail

Preparation time

35 minutes

INGREDIENTS

- 5-6 whole cloves

- 3 cups fresh apple cider

- 2 cups orange juice

- 6 tablespoons honey

- 1 tablespoon orange zest

- 1 teaspoon ground nutmeg

- 4 cinnamon sticks

- 6 cups dry red wine

- Orange, apple, and lemon slices, optional garnish

- Cinnamon sticks, optional garnish

Instructions

1. In a large pot, combine all ingredients except for wine and orange slices and bring to boil.

2. Immediately reduce heat and simmer gently for 30 minutes.

3. Strain in mesh strainer and return to pot.

4. Stir in wine.

5. Keep warm until ready to serve and garnish with cinnamon sticks and orange, apple, and lemon slices.

Kale Pesto

Preparation time

15 minutes

INGREDIENTS

- 1 cup chopped kale

- 2 small chives, chopped

- 1 small green onion, chopped

- 2 tablespoons chopped fresh tarragon

- 2 tablespoons chopped fresh Italian parsley

- 1 anchovy fillet (optional)

- 1 clove garlic

- 1 teaspoon lemon juice

- ¼ teaspoon pepper

- 1/8 teaspoon sea salt

- ¼ cup olive oil

Ingredients

1. In a food processor fitted with a blade, puree kale, chives, green onion, tarragon, parsley, anchovy, garlic, lemon juice, pepper, and sea salt.

2. With the food processor running, slowly pour in olive oil. You may need slightly more or slightly less depending on your desired consistency.

3. Transfer to a small bowl or cup.

4. Use immediately.

5. Cover leftovers with plastic wrap and store in the fridge for up to 5 days.

Easy, Healthy Raspberry Chia Jam

Preparation time

20 minutes

INGREDIENTS

- 1½ cups raspberries, strawberries, or blackberries

- 2 tablespoons honey

- 2 tablespoons chia seeds

Ingredients

1. In a small saucepan, cook down the berries on medium heat until they break down, about 5 minutes.

2. Mash the fruit gently in the saucepan and remove from heat.

3. Add in honey (or other sweetener), stirring to combine.

4. Pour in chia seeds and stir gently to combine.

5. Let set for about 5 minutes to thicken.

6. Let cool and transfer to a glass container and refrigerate.

Lebanese-Style Lentil Soup with Swiss Chard and Lemon (Adas b Hamod)

Preparation time

32 minutes

INGREDIENTS

- 3 cups red lentils

- 12 cups water

- 1 large red onion, diced

- 2 small Yukon gold potatoes, diced

- 1 medium zucchini, diced

- 4 cups Swiss chard, chopped

- 1 bunch of cilantro, chopped

- ¼ cup of lemon juice, more to taste

- 1 teaspoon cumin

- Salt and pepper, to taste

Instructions

1. In a large pot, add lentils and water and place on medium heat to boil.

2. In a pan, sauté onions until pink, about 5 minutes.

3. Add chopped Swiss chard and sauté together until chard is wilted, 2-3 minutes.

4. After lentils have cooked about 8 minutes, add onion chard mixture, along with diced potatoes and zucchini to the boiling water.

5. Add salt and pepper to taste.

6. Reduce heat to medium-low, cover the pot, and cook until the potatoes and lentils are completely cooked, about 12 minutes.

7. Add the chopped cilantro. Stir and cook for about 5 minutes.

8. Add lemon juice and cumin before serving.

Lemon Tahini Herb Sauce

Preparation time

5 minutes

INGREDIENTS

- ½ cup tahini

- 1-2 garlic clove, minced

- Juice of 1 small lemon

- ½ cup almond milk

- 2 tablespoons chopped dill

- Sea salt to taste

Instructions

1. Whisk all ingredients and serve.

2. Keeps in the refrigerator for a week.

Plant-Slant Banana Bread

Preparation time

1 hour

INGREDIENTS

- 2 cups whole wheat pastry flour

- 1 teaspoon baking soda

- ½ teaspoon baking powder

- ½ teaspoon salt

- ½ teaspoon cinnamon

- ½ teaspoon apple cider vinegar

- ½ cup soy milk (or other plant-based milk)

- ½ cup coconut sugar or organic cane sugar

- ½ cup unsweetened applesauce

- 1¼ cups mashed bananas (3-4 ripe bananas)

- 1 teaspoon pure vanilla extract

- ½ cup chopped walnuts

- ½ cup dark chocolate chips, optional

Instructions

1. Preheat the oven to 350 degrees.

2. Prepare a standard size loaf pan by lining it with parchment paper. You can also use 4 mini loaf pans. Very lightly rub cooking spray on them with a paper towel.

3. Pour the soy or almond milk into a bowl and add the apple cider vinegar. Set aside.

4. In a large bowl, mix together the flour, baking soda, baking powder, salt, and cinnamon.

5. Whisk to combine dry ingredients.

6. In the bowl with the soy milk, add the applesauce, sugar, mashed banana, and vanilla extract. Mix well.

7. Add the wet ingredients to the dry ingredients and stir with a rubber spatula until just mixed.

8. Don't overmix.

9. Fold in the walnuts and dark chocolate, if using.

10. Pour the batter into the prepared pan(s).

11. Sprinkle with extra chopped walnuts.

12. Bake at 350 degrees for 35-40 minutes for the standard size pan, or 25-30 minutes for the mini loaf pans, or until a toothpick comes out clean when inserted in the middle.

13. Cool on a wire rack and remove from pan after 15 minutes.

Heirloom Bean Salad with Smoky Sun-Dried Tomato Vinaigrette

Preparation time

2 hours

INGREDIENTS

- 2 cups grated Brussels sprouts

- 1 cup tri-color or red quinoa

- 5 whole bay leaves

- 3 tablespoons sea salt

- 2 tablespoons mushroom base

- 1 tablespoon thyme

- Cilantro, parsley, or fresh scallion, to garnish

SMOKY VINAIGRETTE INGREDIENTS

- 1 cup grapeseed oil

- ½ cup sun-dried tomato

- ⅓ cup white balsamic vinegar

- 2 tablespoons smoked paprika

- 2 tablespoons honey

- 1 tablespoon ground basil

- 1 tablespoon ground black pepper

Instructions

1. Soak legumes for 8 hours prior to cooking.

2. Cook quinoa by boiling in 1 quart of water with mushroom base until the quinoa sprouts. Strain excess liquid and spread onto a baking sheet to cool.

3. Cook legumes for 1½-2 hours in one gallon of rapidly boiling water with sea salt, thyme, and bay leaves, skimming foam occasionally. The largest legumes should be al dente. Strain excess liquid and spread onto a baking sheet to cool.

4. Layer ingredients in a large glass or bowl: quinoa, then grated brussels sprouts, then legumes.

SMOKY VINAIGRETTE DIRECTIONS

1. In a food processor or heavy duty blender, process sun-dried tomato with grapeseed oil until smooth.

2. Add white balsamic vinegar to the tomato-oil mixture and process until emulsified.

3. Add honey, sea salt, ground basil, ground black pepper, and smoked paprika and process until evenly distributed.

4. Drizzle 2 tablespoons of the vinaigrette mixture onto the salads; preserve the rest for future use. Garnish with cilantro, parsley, or fresh scallion (optional).

Dan's Longevity Dal Palak (Spinach Dal)

Preparation time

35 minutes

INGREDIENTS

- 1 cup lentils

- 1 teaspoon garam masala

- 1 teaspoon turmeric

- 1 teaspoon salt

- 1 can (15 ounces) chopped tomatoes

- ⅓ cup oil

- 1 onion, chopped

- 4 – 5 cloves garlic, separated, chopped finely

- 1 inch ginger root, chopped

- 1 teaspoon red pepper flakes

- 1 cup spinach

- 2½ cups water

- Salt to taste

Instructions

1. Sauté all spices and vegetables, except spinach, until onions are clear.

2. Add tomatoes, lentils, and water and simmer for 30 mins.

3. Add spinach and cook for 3 more minutes.

4. Salt to taste.

5. Serve over rice or, if you want an extra longevity boost, use riced cauliflower.

Watermelon Cake

Preparation time

30 minutes

INGREDIENTS

- Watermelon

- 1–2 nectarines, thinly sliced

- Blueberries

- Skewers, to assemble

Instructions

1. Cut the watermelon into three slices. Make one a little bit larger and wider than the other two.

2. Cut off the peel with a knife.

3. Place the largest, widest slice on a cake platter to form the base.

4. Arrange nectarines on top of the watermelon slice.

5. Place 3–4 skewers upright into the watermelon base.

6. Thread 2–3 blueberries onto each skewer. This will hold up the next layer.

7. Carefully push the next watermelon layer through the skewers.

8. Again arrange the nectarines on top of the watermelon and spear 2-3 blueberries onto each skewer.

9. Push the top watermelon layer through the skewers.

10. Top with nectarine slices or blueberries.

11. Push blueberries onto the skewers to decorate.

Pasta with Broccoli, Basil, and Pine Nuts

Preparation time

25 minutes

INGREDIENTS

- 5 cups broccoli florets

- 12 ounces pasta (rotini or ziti work well)*

- 3 tablespoons olive oil

- 2 garlic cloves, minced

- Sea salt and black pepper to taste

- 1 cup pine nuts

- ½ cup seasoned breadcrumbs

- 2 tablespoons fresh chopped basil (or 1 tablespoon of dried basil)

- Crushed red chili pepper flakes, optional garnish

- Grated cheese, optional garnish

Instructions

1. Cook pasta according to package directions until al dente.

2. Drain, reserving ¼ cup of the pasta water. Do not rinse pasta.

3. Put pine nuts and oil in a large saute pan and heat over medium-low heat.

4. When pine nuts start to become golden, add garlic and heat for 2-3 minutes.

5. Before garlic becomes really brown, add broccoli, turn up heat to medium, and cover the pan.

6. Cook for 3-4 minutes until broccoli is cooked but not mushy.

7. Season liberally with salt and pepper and mix to combine.

8. Add pasta to broccoli pan and mix to combine.

9. Turn off heat and add breadcrumbs and basil, stirring to combine.

10. Serve with chili flakes and grated vegetarian cheese, if using.

11. *Note: Feel free to use any pasta you like or use (e.g. bean or lentil pasta, whole-wheat pasta, gluten-free pasta).

Ulu Curry Corn Chowder

Preparation time

30 minutes

INGREDIENTS

- 2 tablespoons extra virgin olive oil

- ¼ teaspoon coriander seeds

- ½ white onion, diced

- 2 cloves garlic

- ¼ teaspoon yellow curry powder

- 1 cup corn

- 2 cups coconut milk

- 1 cup precooked ʻulu (Hawaiian breadfruit)*

- Sea salt, to taste

- ¼ cup water

Instructions

1. Heat oil in a skillet on medium heat and add coriander seeds.

2. Sauté seeds until fragrant.

3. Add onions and garlic and sauté until almost tender.

4. Turn heat up to high and add yellow curry powder, corn, coconut milk, and 'ulu.

5. Bring to a boil and then turn down and let simmer on medium-low until sauce begins to thicken and 'ulu is tender.

6. Add water if sauce thickens too much for your taste.

7. Finish with sea salt and serve.

8. *Note: If 'ulu is not available, use jackfruit, diced sweet potatoes, or another starchy vegetable.

Pineapple Horchata

Preparation time

30 minutes

INGREDIENTS

- 1 pineapple

- 5 cups water

- 1 cup long-grain white rice

- 1 cinnamon stick

- Sugar to taste

Instructions

1. Peel and core the pineapple; reserve the flesh for garnish.

2. Place rice, cinnamon stick, pineapple peels and core with water in a pot; bring to a boil, then lower heat and simmer for 25 minutes.

3. Remove cinnamon stick, peel, and core.

4. Blend in a blender or with an immersion blender.

5. Strain if you want a smooth texture.

6. Add sugar and water if needed, for taste and consistency

7. Garnish with sliced pineapple pieces.